The Advantages of the Clean Diet Plan

Getting Back to a Healthier Lifestyle

By: Amy Zulpa

TABLE OF CONTENTS

Publishers Notes 3

Dedication 4

Chapter 1- What Is Clean Eating? 5

Chapter 2- What Are the Benefits of Eating Clean? 10

Chapter 3- How to Plan Grocery Lists and Meal Plans When Eating Clean? 15

Chapter 4- How to Maintain the Clean Diet in an Unclean World 20

Chapter 5- 10 Clean Eating Breakfast Recipes 25

Chapter 6- 10 Clean Eating Lunch Recipes 36

Chapter 7- 10 Clean Eating Dinner Recipes 49

About the Author 56

Publishers Notes

Disclaimer

This publication is intended to provide helpful and informative material. It is not intended to diagnose, treat, cure, or prevent any health problem or condition, nor is intended to replace the advice of a physician. No action should be taken solely on the contents of this book. Always consult your physician or qualified health-care professional on any matters regarding your health and before adopting any suggestions in this book or drawing inferences from it.

The author and publisher specifically disclaim all responsibility for any liability, loss or risk, personal or otherwise, which is incurred as a consequence, directly or indirectly, from the use or application of any contents of this book.

Any and all product names referenced within this book are the trademarks of their respective owners. None of these owners have sponsored, authorized, endorsed, or approved this book.

Always read all information provided by the manufacturers' product labels before using their products. The author and publisher are not responsible for claims made by manufacturers.

© 2013

Manufactured in the United States of America

Dedication

This book is dedicated to my supportive family.

Chapter 1 - What Is Clean Eating?

The most important aspect of clean eating is eating food that is in its natural state. Clean eating is NOT dieting. Let me repeat...Clean eating is not being on a diet! It is more of a lifestyle choice. Clean eating takes on a different preparation of food and an improved style of eating healthy. An individual that wants to start clean eating has to follow certain steps.

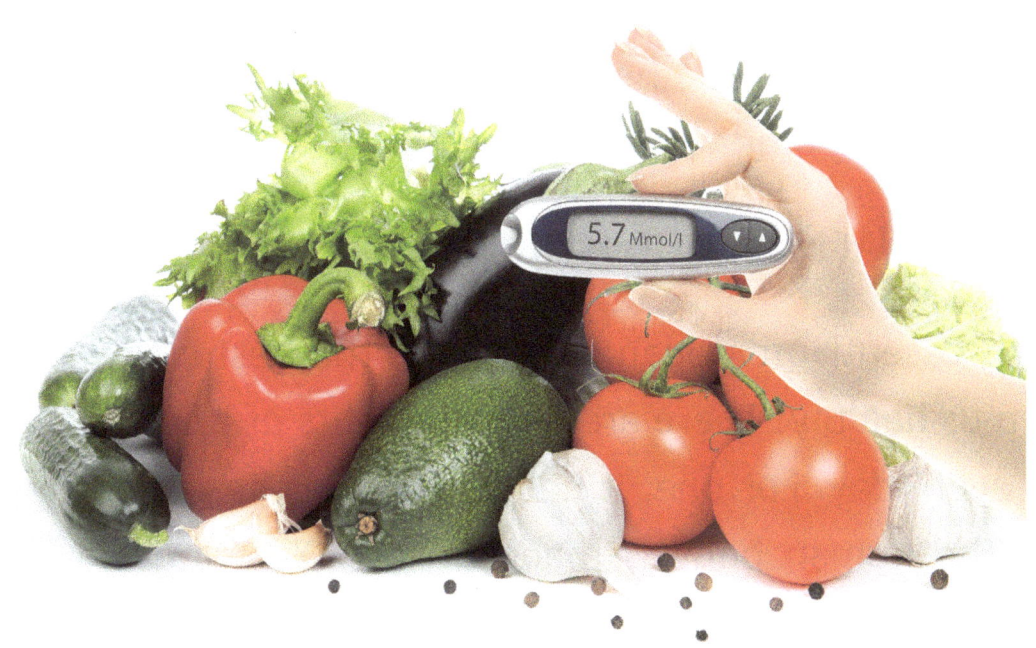

Step 1: Eat 5-6 Times per Day

A lot of people that want to "lose weight" or "eat healthy" either eat significantly less, count calories, or diet. Eating less is not always a good thing though. Starving yourself or consuming only a small amount of calories to lose weight is very unhealthy because your stomach starts to wonder when it is going to get its next meal and stores fat in the mean time. You can imagine that this counterproductive when an individual is trying to be healthy or lose weight.

A much healthier choice would be clean eating and daily exercise. So, eat three decent sized meals and two small snacks. Each meal should include a lean protein, fresh fruit and vegetables, and a complex carbohydrate. By sticking to this routine, your body will stay energized and will keep burning calories all day long. This is much better than starving your stomach and then end up breaking your "diet" because you do not feel satisfied. That just becomes a vicious circle because your body needs nutrition and cannot go a long time without it.

Step 2: Drink At Least 2 Liters of Water per Day

Water is essential for clean eating. It is the best source we have to keep us healthy! There are many benefits of drinking plenty of water every day. For one, it helps maintain the balance of body fluids. The human body is made up of 60% water so you can imagine that giving back what your body is actually made up of is beneficial. Water also helps control calories. It has been proven that it has a weight loss effect because you will be replacing high calorie filled sodas or drinks with water. It also helps fill you up more throughout the day so you will not get any temptations. Why do you think we crave water when exercising or doing physical activities? It is because water helps energize muscles. There are many other benefits of drinking water but to be said, last but not least, it keeps your skin healthy! It has been proven that people that drink more water have healthier and more beautiful looking skin.

Step 3: Read the Labels

Clean foods usually only contain 1-2 ingredients. So, reading the labels is a big one! Those foods that have a huge list of ingredients are man-made and are a big no-no. When clean eating, labels are your best friend.

Step 4: No-No's

Processed foods include anything with flour, sugar, pasta, or bread. We all love these foods so when clean eating, definitely stay away from these! A replacement is a complex carbohydrate such as whole grains. Also keep clear of any foods containing saturated fats and trans fats or anything fried or containing high amounts of sugar.

Step 5: Be Aware

Be aware of fake meats. When shopping for meat, make sure you are buying humanely raised meats and local meats.

Step 6: Go Organic

Whenever possible, eat organically. Unfortunately, organic food can be expensive so when on a budget, make eggs, meat, fruits, vegetables, or dairy.

Step 7: Healthy Fats

Believe it or not, there are such things as "healthy fats." Always choose to consume EFA's or essential fatty acids over unhealthy fats.

Step 8: Portion Sizes

Decent sized meals do not mean big sized meals. Learn to compromise because, again, this does not mean starving your stomach or overeating. Make sure to keep within your portion sizes per meal.

Step 9: Avoid Carbon

Always eat your fruits and vegetables that are in season and grown locally. This effects your expenses and our environment so win-win for the both of you.

Step 10: Don't Rush When Eating

Slow down when consuming each meal. Food tastes better when you are enjoying it! Because of this, you are more satisfied and less tempted.

Step 11: Try Not To Eat Out

In restaurants, you might not always know what is on your plate. When you buy your own food and cook at home, you are staying conscience of what you are consuming. Just because you go to work or school, doesn't mean you have to go get a "quick" bite at lunch. Pack a cooler or lunch bag so you can always eat clean even on the go!

Step 12: Include Your Family or Friends

Since the beginning of time, food has always brought people together. Clean eating will be a lot easier if you are doing it with other people! You will not only be improving your life, but you will be improving other lives as well.

Follow these steps and you will be on your way to a much better and healthier lifestyle. It might be difficult at first but trust me it will be worth it! It will make you happier, more energized, less stressed, and actually makes you feel clean and purified.

Chapter 2 - What Are the Benefits of Eating Clean?

Most diets concentrate on losing weight. However, clean eating is more than just a diet. It is a lifestyle. While weight management (loosing or gaining, based on your individual needs) may be one benefit of clean eating it is definitely not the only reason people are choosing to change their eating habits to include more whole foods and fewer processed foods. There are many physical, mental, social and emotional benefits to clean eating.

Physical Benefits

Weight Management

Because this is the top reason that many people look into various dietary changes it needs to be included. Clean eating helps to control weight gain and weight loss. Many people have large fluctuations in their weight levels over short periods of time. This is often caused by attempting to diet, stress eating, depression, or just being unaware of your dietary habits. Clean eating raises your awareness levels and helps you to eat consistently which stabilizes your weight.

A Healthy Immune System

Since clean eating involves eating whole, unprocessed foods it usually consists of a diet higher in both macro and micro nutrients. The calories you ingest on a clean diet are more efficient at supplying your body with the materials it needs to stay healthy and strong.

A Healthy Cardiovascular System

Clean eating can help you reduce your cholesterol levels and prevent heart disease.

Mental Benefits

Stress management. Clean eating may seem like a lot of work at first. As you take the time to educate yourself about your food options and make changes in your diet you may find yourself more stressed out than you were initially. However, the control that you have over your diet will ultimately lower your stress levels. You will find that having a healthy relationship with food helps to eliminate guilt and stress about your appearance and eating habits.

Higher Energy Levels

The nutrients you get from clean eating such as B-vitamins and iron are more thoroughly absorbed into your system when they are delivered via whole foods as opposed to supplements. These nutrients help you maintain consistent energy levels throughout the day. Normally you may find yourself crashing shortly after a meal that is high in processed foods. Clean eating gives you the proper amount of energy to burn in between smaller meals.

Higher Concentration Levels

Clean eating can help keep your mind clear, allowing you to focus on the important things in your life. The proper balance of proteins and Omegas in your diet can help you concentrate and improve your memory.

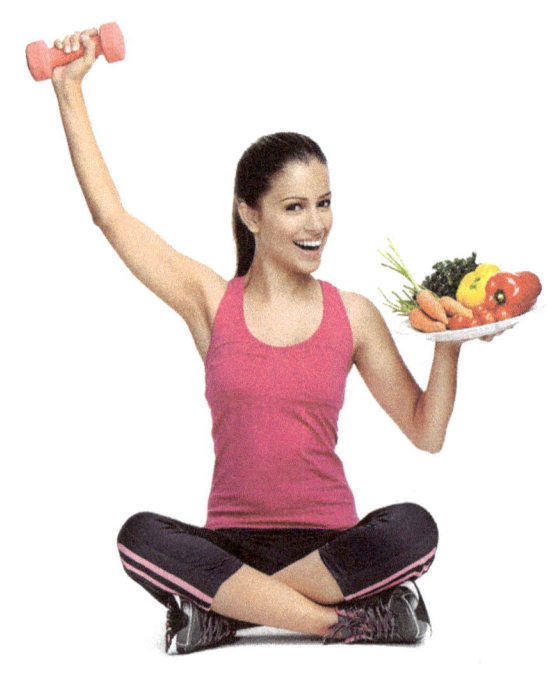

Social Benefits

A Closer Familial Relationship

Many people find that clean eating involves more cooking at home and discussions about food with their family. Some families choose to grow a garden to support their clean eating. These are all activities that can lead to closer familial bonds.

Confidence around Others

As you change your eating habits you will find yourself with more energy and feeling better about how you look. This can help to give you confidence around coworkers, friends, and potential partners.

Opportunities to Make New Friends

People tend to bond over their eating habits. You may find yourself joining a community garden or taking a cooking class to help kick off your clean eating diet. These are great places to meet like-minded people and make new, healthy friends.

Emotional Benefits

Avoid Mood Swings

Mood swings throughout the day are often caused by fluctuating blood-sugar levels. By eating whole foods in smaller portions throughout the day you are allowing your body to avoid spikes in blood-sugar which stabilizes your mood.

Combat Depression

Depression is becoming more and more common these days. One of the reasons for depression is a poor diet. Clean eating increases your absorption of vital vitamins such as B-6 which allow you to produce the chemicals you need to stay happy and alert throughout the day.

A Sense of Control

For people who are overwhelmed with life and feel like there is too much out of their control being educated and aware of their food decisions may help increase their feelings of control. Clean eating involves critical thinking and planning, skills which can be applied to other areas of your life once you have mastered them through your diet.

A Sense of Pride or Accomplishment

Many people struggle with their diet for their entire life. They attempt to, "eat healthy," by following strict regimes and often end up failing. Clean eating allows for many food options and depends on education and awareness rather than unreasoned self-control. For this reason it is easier to be successful following a clean eating diet. That success may increase your confidence and provide you with a feeling of accomplishment.

Clean eating is not a cure-all diet. It is a lifestyle that requires dedication and a large initial commitment of time and energy. However, the benefits of clean eating make that investment worthwhile. One of the best parts of clean eating is its flexibility. You can maintain a clean eating diet and focus on your personal problem areas. If you want to see the physical benefits you can concentrate on portion size. If you want to see the mental benefits you can concentrate on balancing your intake of various nutrients. Whatever you focus on you will still reap many benefits that you aren't even trying to achieve.

Chapter 3- How to Plan Grocery Lists and Meal Plans When Eating Clean?

Seventy percent of the groceries available in supermarkets are chock-full of saturated fats, sodium and sugar and provide little to no nutritional value. For decades, our society eagerly accepted these foods as the nutritional staples for our dinner tables. Society has been conditioned to eat for convenience rather than nutrition. Many of these foods look, smell and even taste good but the truth is there is very little "good for you" in them.

Recently, there has been a growing trend of people becoming more conscious of their health and the foods they consume. By now, you have come to understand the value in foods labeled organic, free-range and fair-trade. You have made the decision to start living a healthy lifestyle beginning with your nutrition. You are ready to clean out the cupboards and fridge to begin stocking your kitchen with fresh, clean foods but one question is plaguing your thoughts...

"How do I shop for clean foods to prepare nutritious meals?"

Changing your lifestyle to include clean, healthy nutrition does not mean that you have to sacrifice your favorite foods. You can continue to enjoy most of the foods you eat now. The difference will be how you start eating the foods you enjoy. When you make the commitment to eating clean foods, you will experience new flavors that should have always existed in your favorite dishes sans preservatives, additives and chemicals. Let's put this in perspective using a food that everyone enjoys- a cookie. Here is a healthy recipe for homemade Oatmeal Raisin Cookies:

Ingredients

2 cups organic oats

1 cup + 2 tablespoons unbleached flour

1 teaspoon ground cinnamon

1/2 teaspoon baking powder

1/2 teaspoon sea salt

1 cup organic sugar

1/3 cup coconut oil, at room temperature

1/3 cup unsweetened applesauce

1 egg

1 teaspoon pure vanilla

1/2 cup raisins

Pre-heat the oven to 350 degrees. Combine ingredients in a large bowl and stir until thoroughly mixed. Drop spoonfuls of dough on a parchment paper lined cookie sheet. Cookies should be placed about 2 inches apart. Gently press cookies to about a ¼ inch in thickness. Bake for 12-14 minutes. Cookies will be soft while cooling.

Now, let's look at the ingredients listed on a common pre-packaged oatmeal cookie: Enriched flour, fortified vitamins, sugar, soybean and palm oil, whole grain oats, raisin paste, baking soda, salt, artificial flavors, cinnamon, propylene glycol alginate, whey, eggs and soy lecithin.

It is clear by the ingredients listed in the homemade recipe what you are putting in your body. However, the prepackaged list of ingredients is confusing and vague. What exactly is contained in the artificial flavors listed? We simply do not know. Yet, millions of these prepackaged cookies are consumed each year.

The first step in changing your eating habits will be meal planning. Begin with outlining two weeks of meals and snacks. If you have a family with children, take into account what everyone enjoys; it is easy to become overzealous and want to perform an overhaul of what everyone has been eating. Remember though, this is about what is in those pizzas, sandwiches and casseroles and not the dishes themselves.

Next, research recipes to prepare the meals you have planned. If you are using the internet to research recipes, it is best to avoid ones that are provided by manufacturers, they often include ingredients that you are trying to eliminate from your diet. It is okay to be adventurous and try a recipe that offers a new twist to an old favorite. As you remove processed foods from your diet, you will find that your taste buds will change and adding new flavors will make the transition more pleasurable.

Finally, it is time to put together your shopping list. Now that you have your recipes, you know the ingredients you will need to purchase. The confusion in clean eating is not what to buy, but learning how to buy. It is easy to be fooled by products labeled as low-fat, whole grain or cholesterol free. The truth is manufacturers use these terms to entice, while barely meeting the minimum requirements set by the FDA.

The information you are looking for is on the back of the product, listed in the ingredients. For instance, a jar labeled "Pure Honey" appears to be a clean food and offer nutrition. However, when you look on the back of the ingredients, it may contain corn syrup, artificial colors and flavors. When choosing a honey there should be three words in the ingredients: Raw, unfiltered honey. Here is your new rule of thumb: Clean foods usually consist of one to six items in the ingredients.

Tips for Choosing Clean Foods

Meats and Fish

Grass-fed and free-range
No Antibiotics
No color added
No water or additional flavors added
No preservatives added

Grains

1 gram of fiber per 10 grams of carbohydrates
No corn syrups
No added colors

No added flavors

No fortified vitamins

No added preservatives

Dairy

Avoid low-fat and fat-free labels

No antibiotics

Organic

Hormone-free

Block cheeses only

No ultra-pasteurized

No added color

No added flavors

No fortified vitamins

Fruits and Vegetables

Organic

As you are transitioning into a healthier lifestyle you are adapting to investing more time into your health. It may seem a bit overwhelming at first, but as you become accustomed to preparing nutritious meals you will realize the benefits to a healthier lifestyle. Soon you will be enjoying foods that you may have previously not liked, as your taste buds and body adapt to clean foods. Good nutrition creates a balanced body, better brain function and emotional stability. You are on the path to a better life, bon appétit!

Chapter 4 - How to Maintain the Clean Diet in an Unclean World

As mentioned beforehand, after choosing to maintain a clean diet you may find yourself wondering just how you can accomplish such a great task. In the modern world there are many obstacles to eating clean including social pressures to consume fast, processed foods, lack of access to clean foods, and lack of time or education concerning clean foods. Instead of becoming overwhelmed with the complexities of eating clean in an unclean world it is important that you have a plan to take control from the beginning.

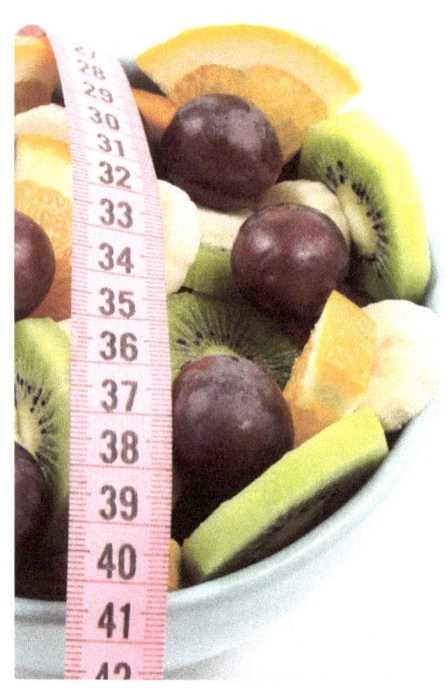

Start Slow

Many people successfully switch to a clean eating regime overnight. However, just as many people struggle for the first couple of months figuring out how to navigate the world of prepackaged food and the need for quick calories in a healthy way. It is important that you allow yourself to make mistakes while learning and changing your diet. Here are some ideas for what you can do to get started that do not involve a radical, overnight change:

Get to know your current habits. Keep a food diary for a week or a month. Write down what you eat, when. Start to realize when you go out to eat and when you cook at home. Do you tend to eat more unprocessed foods at home or while out? How can you increase the amount of whole foods you are eating in these two situations?

Take a look in your pantry. Read the labels of foods you have already purchased. How many of these foods are whole foods and which can be replaced with cleaner options? Make a list of the foods you need to replace and start thinking of substitutes for them before you go shopping.

Concentrate on your options. Many people make the mistake of concentrating on what foods they should avoid. This can be stressful in the beginning. Instead, try making lists of foods that you enjoy that are considered clean. It is easiest to start by simply increasing your fresh fruit and vegetable intake as opposed to buying canned fruits and vegetables. From there you can try more complex substitutions.

Find Support

Many people do not maintain a clean eating diet. While these are still good people it may be difficult to go out with them and resist getting a beer or filling up on empty calories at the bar after work. If you surround yourself with other people who are trying to eat clean you will find it easier to resist temptation. Getting to know other people who are choosing to make clean eating a priority in their lives helps to normalize your choice, giving you greater confidence in your ability to achieve your goals. Plus, you can share your knowledge and tricks for eating clean when you do go out.

Join a community garden. Not everyone who gardens eats clean, but many people interested in gardening do have healthier eating habits than the average person. At a community garden you not only gain access to a variety of fresh, whole foods but you can also meet interesting people who share your values regarding food.

Get your family on board. It is difficult to change your eating habits when the rest of your family wants to continue eating the way they always have. Try to get your family excited about the benefits of clean eating. Make food a central part of your family life. The support of those closest to you can often make or break your commitment to your new lifestyle.

Find a clean eating cooking class. A great way to meet people who have the same values as you is to take a class with them. Not only will you learn recipes and different methods for healthy food preparation but you will also begin to develop a support network.

Prepare Your Own Food

Many people think that clean eating has to be time consuming because your choices of food become limited. It is true that prepackaged food is quick, but there are many quick and easy recipes for clean eating that do not take much longer than stopping at the drive-thru on the way home from work. Preparing your own food allows you to have greater control over your diet and to know exactly what ingredients are going into your meals. Although there are many options for dining out, most people find it easier to maintain clean eating at home.

Host clean eating picnics. Just because you are eating clean does not mean you should abstain from the social culture built around food. People enjoy themed barbecues or picnics. Try hosting a clean eating picnic, perhaps making it a regular event.

Cook in advance. If you have a free weekend you can prepare your lunches in advance. Chop fruits and vegetables and make a few bulk dishes that you can easily pack for work.

Make food fun. If cooking and eating becomes a source of entertainment for you and your family it is more likely that you will make time for it. Make food preparation a fun, family event or use the time alone to unwind from a busy day.

Eating healthy in a culture that idolizes fast, unhealthy food choices can be difficult. However, it is not impossible. With a few lifestyle changes eating healthy will become second nature.

Chapter 5- 10 Clean Eating Breakfast Recipes

Since we were children, we have been told that breakfast is the most important meal of the day. Breakfast gives us the nutrients and the energy that we need to get through the day. When choosing a breakfast dish, it is a good idea to find a "clean" breakfast dish. Clean breakfast dishes are excellent for those trying to eat healthy and get fit.

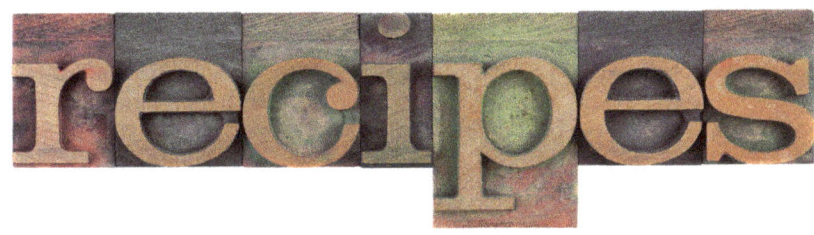

Cheesy Potato Frittata

This is an excellent clean breakfast dish. It is less than 200 calories and has just 4 grams of fat. You can't go wrong with that.

Ingredients

8 medium potatoes
1 egg
2 tablespoons of skim milk
6 egg whites
1/4 cup of fresh parsley
1 ½ cups yellow onion
1 clove of garlic

2 ounces of low fat, extra sharp cheddar cheese

1/2 cup of sour cream (low fat)

1 teaspoon of salt, divided

1 teaspoon of pepper

1 teaspoon of sesame oil

Directions

Begin by preparing your ingredients. Scrub the potatoes well and cut them into ½ inch cubes. Next chop the parsley and the onion. Finally, mince the garlic.

Put 2 cups of water on in a medium pot and let come to a boil. Add the potatoes and allow them to boil. Reduce heat to medium and allow them to cook until they are tender (about twelve minutes). Using a colander, drain the potatoes and set them aside.

In a bowl, add the parsley, milk, egg whites, egg and ¼ teaspoon of salt. Use a whisk and blend the ingredients until fully incorporated. Once mixed, set aside.

Heat the oil in a large skillet. Once heated, add the onions. Stir them occasionally, cooking until the edges are brown. Next add the garlic. Cook for about 15 seconds and stir constantly. Next, put in the potatoes and keep stirring until are the ingredients are mixed completely and reduce the heat to low. Next, whisk the egg mixture over the potato mixture very slowly. Be sure that you distribute it evenly so that all the potatoes are covered. Cover the skillet and allow to cook for about 12 minutes or until the egg mixture is nearly set and take it off the heat. Top the dish with the remaining salt and the cheddar cheese. Cover and let stand for about 15 minutes to give the cheese a chance to melt. Cut the frittata into 4 wedges and put sour cream on top of each wedge.

Minty Citrus Breakfast Salad

This is an amazing clean breakfast. It is not only delicious; it is also very low in fat.

Ingredients

1 orange
1 pink grapefruit
2 mandarin oranges
4 kumquats
1 lime
2 tablespoons of finely chopped fresh mint leaves

Directions

Begin by peeling the oranges and the grapefruit. Pull them apart in wedges and cut the wedges into bite sized pieces. Place all of these ingredients in a bowl. Next, cut away the peel of the citrus. Using a paring knife, cut in between the membranes to remove the fruit segments and add them to the bowl. Next cut the kumquats and add them to the bowl along with the mint. Combine until the salad is fully incorporated. Place in the refrigerator for about 15 minutes before serving. This breakfast salad will make 4 servings. If you keep it refrigerated, it should keep for about a week.

Vegetarian Hash

This is an excellent dish loaded with nutrients. The acorn squash in this breakfast has more potassium than a banana.

Ingredients

3/4 pounds of small potatoes
1 acorn squash
2 cups of broccoli
1/3 cup red pepper
1/3 cup green pepper
1/2 teaspoon salt
1/2 teaspoon pepper
4 tablespoons of olive oil
2 tablespoon of lemon juice
6 eggs
1/4 cup of skim milk

Directions

Begin by preparing the ingredients. Wash the potatoes. If they are too large, you may want to cut them in half. Next peel and cut the acorn squash and cut it into ¼ inch pieces. Take the broccoli and shred it. Break the eggs over a bowl and whisk the eggs and the milk. Finally, slice the 2 peppers very thin.

Preheat your oven to 425 degrees. In a large bowl, mix the potatoes, acorn squash, ½ teaspoon of salt, and ¼ teaspoon of pepper. On a large baking sheet, spray cooking spray and pour the mixture on the baking sheet. Pour 2 tablespoons of olive oil over the entire mixture and gently toss. Bake in the oven for about 25 minutes or until the potatoes and acorn squash are tender while stirring every 10 minutes and remove from the oven.

In a large skillet, heat the remaining oil until hot. Add the peppers and the broccoli and sauté for 3 minutes. Add the potato mixture to the skillet and mix until fully incorporated. Allow to cook for about 5 minutes.

Using a spatula, push all of the food to one side of the pan. Pour the eggs on the other side of the pan. Allow them to cook until they are no longer wet while stirring constantly. When the eggs are done, mix them in with the potato mixture. Serve while still hot.

Amazing Breakfast Frittata

This dish is delicious and it is good for you. It is low fat and can be whipped up in 15 minutes making it an excellent dish to make before work.

Ingredients

8 egg whites. If you are using the egg whites in a carton, use 1 cup
1 egg with the yolk
1/3 cup of skim milk
2/3 cups of skim ricotta cheese
2 cups of baby spinach
2 cups of kale
2 cloves of garlic
1 onion
1 tablespoon of olive oil
1/4 teaspoon of salt
1/4 teaspoon of pepper

Directions

Begin by preparing your ingredients. Slice the onion thin, mince the garlic, and rip the kale bunch in half. . In a bowl, whisk the egg whites, egg, and the milk until fully incorporated and set all the ingredients aside.

Heat the oil in a skillet over a medium flame. Add the onion and garlic and sauté for about 3 minutes or until they have softened. Add the spinach and the kale to the pan and cook until they start to wilt. Stir in the pepper and salt. Put the egg mixture in the pan and drop the ricotta cheese over the mixture tablespoon by tablespoon and cook for about 3 minutes or until the eggs start to set. Place the pan in the oven at 375 degrees and bake for about

8 minutes or until the eggs are firm. Remove from the oven and cut into 4 wedges. Serve while hot.

Coconut Mango Oatmeal

This is an excellent breakfast which tastes great and is good for you. This dish needs to chill overnight; therefore, you need to prepare it the night before.

Ingredients

1/2 cup of oatmeal
1/2 cup of almond milk
1/2 cup of mango
1 tablespoon of shredded coconut

Directions

Begin by chopping the mango into small, bite sized pieces. In a jar with a cover, mix all of the ingredients until fully incorporated. Cover and refrigerate overnight. In the morning, enjoy.

Super Breakfast Pocket

This dish contains clean super foods and tastes amazing. It is great when you need to eat on the run.

Ingredients

2 eggs
2 egg whites

1 tablespoon of skim milk

1 cup of baby spinach

4 grape tomatoes

2 small onions

¼ cup feta cheese crumbles

Dash of salt

Dash of pepper

2 teaspoons of olive oil

Whole wheat pita pocket cut in half

Directions

Begin by preparing the ingredients. Tear the spinach into small pieces, and slice the tomatoes in half. In a mixing bowl, whisk together the egg whites, eggs, skim milk, spinach, tomatoes, onions, and salt and pepper. Pour the mixture into an oven safe baking dish at 350 degrees. Cook for about 15 minutes or until it is fluffy and just set in the middle then brush both sides of the pita with the olive oil. Wrap it in aluminum foil. Place it in the oven during the last 2 minutes of baking the egg mixture. Remove the baking dish and the pita bread from the oven. Cut the egg mixture in half and place each in the pocket.

Super Clean Smoothie

If you prefer a quick but filling smoothie for breakfast, this is the smoothie for you. It contains all of the clean foods that your body needs to get it started for your day.

Ingredients

1 small banana

1 cup of baby spinach

1 cup of blueberries (frozen)

1/2 cup of plain, low fat, Greek yogurt

1/2 cup of pomegranate juice

1 cup of chilled, unsweetened green tea

1 cup of crushed ice

Directions

Before you prepare your smoothie, it is necessary to slice the banana and place it in the freezer. Let it stay in there for about an hour or until frozen.

Take all of the ingredients and place them in the blender. Blend for about 1 minute and pour in a glass. Enjoy.

Cleanest Grits

This is an excellent dish which can be prepared in about 20 minutes. It is made in single servings and can be eaten on the run.

Ingredients

2 teaspoons of maple syrup

1 cup skim milk

1/4 cup of instant grits

2 tablespoons of raisins

Dash of salt

Directions

In a small sauce pan, bring the milk, syrup and salt to a boil. Whisk the grits in slowly whisk and reduce heat to medium low. Cover and continue to cook for about 3 minutes. Take it off the heat and let sit for 1 minute. Sprinkle the raisins over the top, mix them in if desired.

Berry Pomegranate Smoothie

This is a clean smoothie if you need to have breakfast on the run. When it is done, simply pour in a travel cup and go. It will give you the same nutrients you would get from a big breakfast.

Ingredients

2 cups of frozen raspberries
1/2 cup of water
1/2 cup skim cottage cheese
1 banana
1 cup of pomegranate juice

Directions

Add the ingredients to the blender. Blend until consistency is smooth. Serve immediately while still cold.

Granola Mix

This is an excellent granola recipe. It is cleaner than a store bought granola bar and tastes better too.

Ingredients

5 cups of oats
1/2 cups of pecans
1/2 cups of almonds
1/3 cups of pumpkin seeds
1/2 cups of dried cranberries
1/2 cups of raisins
1/2 cups of brown sugar
½ cups of maple syrup
1/4 cups of canola oil
1/2 cups of water
1 cup of coconut flakes

Directions

Begin by preparing the ingredients. Slice the almonds thinly and coarsely chop the pecans. In a big bowl, mix the sunflower seeds, pumpkin, brown sugar, pecans, almonds coconut and oats.

In a separate bowl, combine the oil, water and syrup. Pour over the mixture and stir until fully incorporated. On a large baking sheet with a rim, spread the mixture. Bake for 45 minutes at 275 degrees stirring once halfway through. Cook for 45 minutes longer. Take it from the oven and add the cranberries and the raisins. Allow to cool before storing in a container.

Chapter 6- 10 Clean Eating Lunch Recipes

When trying to eat clean, it can sometimes be difficult. In a fast paced world, many people go out and grab a quick bite on their lunch break. The problem with this is that fast food restaurants do not always have healthiest menu. The best is to make a lunch yourself.

The Cleanest Cobb Salad

This salad is very low in fat. By making your own dressing, you can be sure that it is healthier than the dressings you will buy in the supermarket.

Ingredients

6 cups of chopped romaine lettuce
2 avocados
1 pound of boneless chicken breast
2 tomatoes

Dressing Ingredients:

1/4 cup of red wine vinegar
1/2 cup of olive oil
1 teaspoon of maple syrup
Dash of salt
Dash of pepper

Directions

Begin by preparing your ingredients. In a large bowl, break up the lettuce. Next, peel, seed, and chop the avocado in 1 inch pieces. Cut your tomatoes either in slices or wedges, which ever you prefer. Take your chicken breast and cut it into 1 ½ pieces. In a sauté pan, add a small amount of oil and cook the chicken until it is no longer pink. Be sure to cook the chicken all the way through to prevent salmonella. After the chicken is done, combine all the ingredients with the lettuce. Mix until fully incorporated.

Prepare the dressing by combining all of the ingredients and drizzle over the salad.

This salad will make enough to eat a few days a week for lunch.

Bean and Spinach Burrito Wrap

This is an excellent meal for lunch. It is easily prepared and can conveniently be taken to work in a brown lunch bag.

Ingredients

6 cups of baby spinach
1 ½ cups of brown rice
1 can of black beans
1/2 cup of romaine lettuce
1/2 cup of reduced fat shredded cheddar cheese
1/2 cup of salsa
6 tablespoons of plain, fat free, Greek yogurt
6 whole grain tortillas

Dash of salt

Directions

Begin by preparing the ingredients. Drain and rinse the beans, chop the lettuce, and cook the brown rice.

Preheat the oven to 300 degrees. Wrap the stacked tortillas in aluminum foil. Place them on a cookie sheet and allow them to warm for about 15 minutes.

In a food processor, pulse the spinach until it is finely chopped. If you do not have a food processor, you can use a knife to dice the spinach into very fine pieces. In a large skillet, combine the spinach and the black beans. Cook for about 3 minutes over medium heat or until the spinach wilts.

Remove the tortillas from the oven. Evenly distribute the spinach and bean mixture in the middle of the wrap. Next, add the rice, lettuce, cheese, salsa, and the Greek yogurt over the wrap. Fold the wraps over and under on the ends. This will make 6 burritos. Wrap the burritos that you do not need to take and refrigerate them. They will keep for about 5 days.

Brown Rice and Vegetable Stir Fry

This is a very healthy dish that is great eaten hot or cold. If you have access to a microwave at work, you can heat it. If not, it tastes excellent as a salad. The rice mixture will need to cool for 2 hours before you put the dish together, therefore, you should allow ample time when preparing this dish.

Ingredients

1 cup of brown rice
2 cups of low sodium chicken broth
1 tablespoon of olive oil
1 teaspoon of sesame oil
1 cup of carrots
1/2 cup of green onions
2 cloves of garlic
1/2 cup of frozen peas
2 eggs
Dash of salt
2 tablespoons of gluten free soy sauce

Directions

Begin by preparing the ingredients. Chop the carrots into fine pieces. Chip the green onions and mince the garlic. Allow your peas to thaw and beat the eggs in a small bowl.

In a sauce pan, add the brown rice and the broth. Over medium high heat, bring to a boil. Cover the pan and reduce the heat to a simmer. Allow to cook for about 15 minutes or until the broth has been absorbed by the rice. Remove from the heat and place in the refrigerator and allow to cool for about 2 hours.

In a large skillet, heat the oils over medium heat. Add the carrots and the green onions. Cover the pan and allow to cook until they are tender. This should take about 8 minutes. Add the garlic and continue cooking for another minute. Add the brown rice and peas and cook for 5 minutes.

Push all of the food to the side of the skillet. Add the eggs to the empty side and add the eggs. Scramble until they are no longer runny. When they are done, push the brown rice back over the eggs and stir until they are fully incorporated. Pour the soy sauce over the mixture and cook for about 1 minute.

Clean Eating Superfood Soup

This meal has all of the best clean eating foods. It needs to be made in a crock pot, therefore, it is wise to prepare it the night before. It will need to cook for about 8 hours giving you the chance to prepare it right before bed and it will be ready when you wake up.

Ingredients

2 cups of carrots

1 sweet potato

1 cup of green beans, fresh or frozen

1/2 cup of cilantro

1 small onion

1 clove

2 cans of black beans

2 cups of vegetable juice, use organic with no sugar added

2 cups of low sodium vegetable broth

1/2 teaspoon of red pepper flakes

1/2 teaspoon of black pepper

1 teaspoon of chili powder

1 teaspoon of cumin

Dash of salt

Directions

Begin by preparing your ingredients. Slice the carrots, and the sweet potatoes. Next, chop the cilantro, dice the onion, and mince the garlic.

In a slow cooker, combine all of the ingredients. Cover and cook for about 8 hours or until the vegetables are tender.

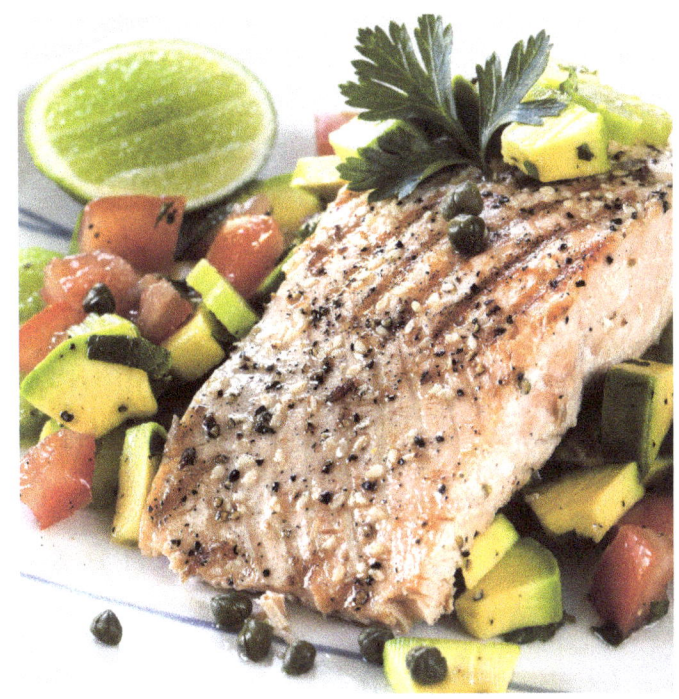

Grilled Shrimp Salad Served in an Avocado Shell

This is a very clean lunch. Because it is served right from an avocado shell, it makes it very handy to take to work every day. The ingredients work together making this a delicious super food.

Ingredients

3 avocados
1 pound of miniature shrimp
1/4 cups of scallions
1 teaspoon of paprika
1 teaspoon of cumin
2 bell peppers
2 tablespoons of lemon juice, split
2 tablespoons of olive oil
1 teaspoon of mustard
1 cup of plain, non fat, Greek yogurt
Dash of salt
Dash of pepper

Directions

Begin by peel the shrimp and remove the claws. In a sauce pan, add some oil and cook the shrimp until cooked through. When it is pink and firm it can be removed from the heat.

Next you want to prepare your dressing. In a small bowl, whisk together the mustard and half of the lemon juice. Continue to whisk while you add the olive oil.

To prepare your peppers, you want to place them in the broiler over high heat. Be sure that the fame is coming in contact directly with the peppers. Allow to cook until one side blackens. Flip and blacken the other side. Next, place the peppers in a zip lock bag and close. This will make peeling the peppers easier.

After 10 minutes, remove the peppers and peel them. First remove the stem and the seeds. Rub the skin with a wet towel and cut them into small strips. For the yogurt topping, combine the yogurt, cumin, paprika add the remaining lemon juice and set aside.

To prepare the avocado shell, take a tablespoon and scoop out the avocado. Be sure that you leave a good amount still inside. Take the avocado that was scooped out and chop into bite sized pieces. To put it all together, combine the avocado pieces, chives, red pepper, shrimp, and the dressing in a large bowl. Mix until it is creamy. Spoon the mixture into the avocado shells for serving.

Greek Yogurt Egg Salad

This is an excellent sandwich that has all of the super foods that you need to eat clean.

Ingredients

1 avocado
2 cups arugula
1 teaspoon of dried dill

2 tomatoes

8 eggs

1 tablespoon of light mayonnaise

2/3 cup of low fat, plain, Greek yogurt

Dash of salt

Dash of pepper

4 whole wheat wraps

Directions

Begin by boiling the eggs. In a large sauce pan, allow them to sit in boiling water for 15 minutes. Carefully remove them, peel and chop them into small pieces. Transfer to a large bowl. Next add the arugula and the chopped avocado and stir in with the eggs. Add the dried dill, mayonnaise, yogurt, and the salt and pepper. Combine until all of the ingredients are fully incorporated. Serve on the whole wheat wraps. If you do not need to use all of the mixture, cover and refrigerate. It should keep for about 5 days.

Asian Pasta Salad

This is an excellent dish. It is delicious and healthy. It is also easy to make and it will make about 4 lunches.

Ingredients

1 avocado

1 carrot

1 green onion

1 mango

1/4 cup of red cabbage

2 tablespoons gluten free soy sauce

8 ounces of elbow pasta

1/2 teaspoons of sesame seeds

1 ½ tablespoons of sugar

Dash of salt

Dash of pepper

2 tablespoons of pine nuts

Directions

Begin by preparing the ingredients. Chop the avocado, carrots, green onion, and mango. Break up the red cabbage into bite sized pieces. Next prepare the pasta according to the directions on the back of the box.

In a large bowl, combine all the ingredients. Stir until it is fully incorporated. Place the dish in the refrigerator for about 2 hours or until cold.

Cleanest Chicken Salad

This is an excellent chicken salad recipe. This can be either served on a whole wheat wrap or over a tossed green salad.

Ingredients

1/2 pound of chicken

1 cup of celery

1 cup of grapes

1/4 cup of green onion

1/2 teaspoon onion powder

1/2 teaspoon of salt

1/2 teaspoon of pepper

1/2 cup of pecans

3/4 cups of light mayonnaise

Directions

Begin by cooking the chicken. Cut it up in a few pieces for faster cooking. Allow to cook until it is cooked through and no longer pink. Next, grate the chicken into small pieces. Transfer them to large bowl.

Next, chop the celery, grapes, and onion into small pieces. Add them in with the chicken. Add the salt, pepper, and onion powder. Chop the pecans into small pieces and add all of these ingredients to the bowl. Finally, add the mayonnaise. Stir until the ingredients are fully incorporated. Place in the refrigerator for about 2 hours or until cold.

Avocado and Cucumber Sandwich

This is a very healthy dish that is very simple to make. If you are running late for work and need to throw together a quick lunch, this one is great.

Ingredients

1 cucumber

1 avocado

Dash of salt

Dash of pepper

Low fat garden style cream cheese

2 slices of whole wheat bread

Directions

Begin by peeling and slicing your cucumber into 12 slices. Next slice the avocado. Put a small thin layer of the cream cheese on each of the slices of bread. Stack the avocado and cucumber and add the salt and pepper to taste.

This recipe will make 1 sandwich. If you want 2 sandwiches, feel free to double the recipe.

Cleanest Tuna Sandwiches

This is an excellent recipe for tuna lovers. It make 4 sandwiches, therefore, you can refrigerate the extra tuna and use another day.

Ingredients

1 can of albacore tuna in water (do not use the tuna in oil)

2 cups of spinach

1/2 cup of red peppers

1/4 cup of onion

1/2 cup of light mayonnaise

8 slices of whole wheat bread

Directions

Begin by preparing your ingredients. Chop the spinach, the red peppers, and the onion. Place them in a large bowl. Open the tuna and drain all of the water. Mix it in with the vegetables. Finally, add the mayonnaise. Mix until it is fully incorporated. Place the bowl, covered, in the refrigerator for about 2 hour or until cold. Leftovers will keep for about 5 days.

CHAPTER 7- 10 CLEAN EATING DINNER RECIPES

Protein Shake

Ingredients

1 cup almond milk
1 scoop whey protein powder
Handful frozen berries
Handful fresh kale
Dash of cinnamon

Directions

The best way to eat clean is to have a protein shake for dinner. Begin by adding a cup of almond milk to your blender, then adding a scoop of your favorite flavor of whey protein powder. Then add the berries and kale, which will an abundance of nutrients. Top the protein shake off with a dash of cinnamon and blend together until smooth.

Quinoa Salad

Ingredients

1 cup quinoa
2 cups water
1 tablespoon olive oil
1/2 cup garbanzo beans
Feta cheese

Cilantro
Salt and pepper

Directions

Begin by adding 2 cups of water and 1 cup of quinoa to a sauce pan on high heat. Once the water comes to a boil, bring the heat down to low for about 15 minutes or until the water is soaked up. Then, place the quinoa in a large mixing bowl and mix in the olive oil, garbanzo beans, and a little feta cheese, cilantro, and salt and pepper, to taste.

Chicken Breast

Ingredients

1 pound chicken breast cutlets
1 tablespoon of coconut oil
Salt and pepper
Garlic powder

Directions

To create another protein-rich clean dinner, begin by adding the coconut oil to a pan over medium heat. After rinsing and patting the chicken dry, add the cutlets to the pan and season with salt, pepper, and a dash of garlic powder. Allow the chicken to cook for about five minutes, and then flip them. Season this side with salt, pepper, and garlic powder and allow to cook for about five minutes. Be sure to check the chicken by cutting down the middle to see if it's fully cooked (no pink in the middle) and cook a little longer on each side, if necessary.

Crock Pot Chili

Ingredients

1 pound of ground beef
1 tablespoon olive oil
3 cans of beans
1 can tomato sauce
1 large carrot, sliced
1 large onion, sliced
2 bell peppers, sliced
2 stalks celery, sliced

Directions

Chili is as healthy as you make it, simply add a wide array of veggies to stock up on vitamins. Begin by browning the beef in an olive oil coated pan over medium heat. While the meat is browning, add the tomato sauce to your crock pot. Then add in the browned beef and whatever veggies and beans you'd like, like garbanzo beans, an onion, a carrot, celery, and bell pepper. Add seasonings of your choice and allow to simmer for several hours.

Chocolate Berry Yogurt

Ingredients

1 cup plain Greek yogurt
1 scoop whey protein powder
1 tablespoon almond butter
1/2 cup frozen berries

Directions

Although this chocolate meal may seem like a dessert, it's actually protein-rich and will satisfy your sweet tooth. Simply add a scoop of whey protein powder to the yogurt, then add a dollop of almond butter. Next, add in the frozen berries, which will freeze immediately upon contact, creating an ice cream-like dessert for dinner.

Mock Potatoes

Ingredients

1 cauliflower head, cut into florets
1 tablespoon olive oil
A few cloves of garlic
Salt and pepper

Directions

While potatoes aren't usually part of a clean eating list, cauliflower makes a great substitute. Begin by steaming cauliflower florets until tender. Once tender, place them into a large mixing bowl and mash them up. Then, add the olive oil, garlic, and salt and pepper to taste.

Spinach Salad

Ingredients:

2 cups spinach
1 tomato, sliced
1 tablespoon olive oil
Goat cheese
Salt and pepper

Directions

Consuming a sufficient amount of greens is imperative when eating clean. To create this spinach salad, begin with your spinach base and add sliced tomato. Then, add goat cheese to taste, drizzle with olive oil, and sprinkle with salt and pepper.

Dried Fruit and Nut Cereal

Ingredients

1 cup almond milk
1/2 cup very thinly sliced almonds
1/2 cup chopped pecans
1 banana, sliced
1/2 cup dried, unsweetened cherries

Directions

Generally, cereal doesn't fall under the clean eating list. Luckily, there is a healthy alternative. Begin by placing the almonds in a cereal bowl with the chopped pecans. Next, add the almond milk and top with banana and cherries, or your favorite dried, unsweetened fruit.

Stuffed Avocados

Ingredients

1 avocado, peeled and pitted
A few tablespoons of ground beef
1 tablespoon olive oil
Salt and pepper

Directions

To create the vitamin-rich meal of stuffed avocados, begin by browning the ground beef in an olive oil coated pan over medium heat. Once brown, simply take one of the avocado halves and stuff with ground beef, salt and pepper to taste, and your favorite seasonings.

Stuffed Bell Pepper

Ingredients

1 large bell pepper
A few tablespoons of ground beef
1 tablespoon olive oil
Salt and pepper

Directions:

Similarly to stuffed avocados, stuffed peppers offer various vitamins and protein. First, cut a square shape in the top of a bell pepper and remove the core. Then, brown the beef in an olive oil coated pan over medium heat, adding salt and pepper to taste. Once brown, stuff the beef into the bell pepper.

ABOUT THE AUTHOR

Amy Zulpa made a big change to her lifestyle when she decided that she simply had to stop eating all of the junk foods that she so loved to consume. It was not that she necessarily wanted to go on a diet but she just wanted to get rid of the foods that were bad for her. She did her research and found that it was not hard to make the transition to the clean eating lifestyle.

It was something that could be done gradually and nothing was wrong if a sweet treat was had from time to time. This is what she started to promote. A diet in the conventional sense was not necessary at all. All that was required to get started on a healthier lifestyle was a change in what was being consumed and the amount that was being consumed.